A 10 Minutes Flexibility Guide

Zena Olson Therapy's Approach For Reduced Pain And Improved Performance And Body Reconstruction Plus Dietary Guide

Zena Olson

Table of Contents

CHAPTER ONE

Introduction

Fitness training and personal coaching play a crucial role in promoting overall well-being and achieving optimal physical health. In today's fast-paced and sedentary lifestyle, where technology often dominates our daily activities, it has become increasingly important to prioritize fitness and take proactive steps towards maintaining a healthy lifestyle.

Regular exercise, combined with personalized coaching and guidance, can have a profound impact on our physical, mental, and emotional well-being. Fitness training helps improve cardiovascular health, increase strength and endurance, enhance flexibility, and manage weight. It also plays a pivotal role in preventing chronic diseases such as obesity, diabetes, and heart conditions.

While the benefits of exercise are widely recognized, many individuals struggle to incorporate regular physical activity into their routines due to various factors, such as lack of motivation, knowledge, or time constraints. This is where personal coaching becomes invaluable. A personal coach provides guidance, support, and expertise to help individuals set and achieve their fitness goals.

Personal coaching goes beyond mere exercise instruction. It involves understanding an individual's unique needs, abilities, and limitations and tailoring a fitness program accordingly. Coaches can help individuals establish realistic goals, develop personalized workout routines, provide nutritional guidance, and offer accountability and motivation throughout the fitness journey.

Furthermore, personal coaches can assist in overcoming barriers and challenges that individuals may face along the way. They can provide guidance on proper exercise techniques, prevent injuries, and adjust training plans to accommodate changing circumstances or physical limitations. Additionally, coaches can offer emotional support, helping individuals stay motivated, overcome self-doubt, and maintain a positive mindset.

In today's interconnected world, personal coaching has become more accessible than ever. With advancements in technology, virtual coaching sessions and online fitness platforms have emerged, allowing individuals to receive personalized guidance and support from the comfort of their homes.

Fitness training and personal coaching are vital components of a healthy lifestyle. They provide individuals with the tools, knowledge, and support they need to embark on a fitness journey, achieve their goals, and maintain long-term well-being. By prioritizing fitness and seeking the guidance of a personal coach, individuals can optimize their physical health, enhance their mental and emotional resilience, and enjoy a higher quality of life.

Your Fitness Goals

Before embarking on any fitness training program, it is crucial to assess and define your fitness goals. Understanding what you want to achieve allows you to tailor your training plan and focus your efforts in the right direction. Here are some steps to help you assess and define your fitness objectives:

1. Self-Reflection: Take some time to reflect on your current fitness level and what aspects of your health and well-being you would like to improve. Consider your strengths, weaknesses, and any specific areas you would like to

target, such as cardiovascular endurance, strength, flexibility, or weight management.

2. Set Specific Goals: Once you have identified the areas you want to work on, set specific and measurable goals. For example, instead of saying, "I want to get fit," define your goal as "I want to be able to run a 5K race within three months." Specific goals provide clarity and help you track your progress effectively.

3. Consider Timeframe: Determine a realistic timeframe for achieving your

goals. Setting a deadline can help you stay focused and motivated. However, be mindful of setting attainable goals that allow for gradual progress and avoid pushing yourself too hard, which can lead to burnout or injury.

4. Make Goals Challenging yet Achievable: It's important to strike a balance between setting challenging goals and ensuring they are attainable. Pushing yourself outside of your comfort zone can lead to significant improvements, but setting unrealistic goals may result in frustration and disappointment. Consider your current fitness level,

available time, and any constraints you may have.

5. Seek Professional Guidance: If you're uncertain about setting appropriate fitness goals or need help assessing your current fitness level, consider consulting with a fitness professional. They can conduct assessments, discuss your objectives, and provide valuable insights and guidance tailored to your needs.

Essential Components of Fitness Training

Once you have defined your fitness goals, it's time to build a solid foundation for your training program. The following components are essential for a well-rounded and effective fitness routine:

1. Cardiovascular Endurance: Cardiovascular exercises such as running, cycling, swimming, or brisk walking help strengthen your heart and lungs, improve circulation, and boost overall endurance. Aim for at least 150 minutes of moderate-intensity aerobic activity or 75 minutes of vigorous-intensity aerobic activity per week.

2. Strength Training: Incorporate strength training exercises to improve muscle

strength, tone, and overall body composition. Use resistance training equipment, free weights, or bodyweight exercises like push-ups, squats, and lunges. Aim for at least two to three strength training sessions per week, targeting different muscle groups.

3. Flexibility and Mobility: Include stretching exercises or activities like yoga or Pilates to improve flexibility, joint range of motion, and posture. These exercises can enhance athletic performance, prevent injuries, and promote better overall movement quality.

4. Balance and Stability: Incorporate exercises that focus on improving balance and stability to reduce the risk of falls, especially as you age. These exercises can include standing on one leg, yoga poses that challenge balance, or specific balance training equipment.

5. Rest and Recovery: Allow for adequate rest and recovery days in your training program. Rest is essential for your muscles to repair and grow stronger. Overtraining can lead to injuries and hinder progress, so listen to your body and give it the time it needs to recover.

Remember that consistency and progression are key when it comes to fitness training. Gradually increase the intensity, duration, or frequency of your workouts as your fitness level improves. Stay motivated by tracking your progress, celebrating milestones, and seeking ongoing support from a personal coach or workout buddy. With a solid foundation and a well-designed training program, you can work towards achieving your fitness goals and enjoy the numerous benefits of a healthy and active lifestyle.

CHAPTER TWO

Cardiovascular Conditioning

Cardiovascular conditioning, also known as aerobic exercise, is essential for improving heart health, increasing stamina, and burning calories. Here are some key points to consider for cardiovascular training:

1. Choose an Activity: Select activities that elevate your heart rate and engage large muscle groups. Running, cycling, swimming, brisk walking, dancing, or participating in aerobic classes are great options. Pick activities that you enjoy to stay motivated.

2. Intensity and Duration: Aim for moderate to vigorous intensity workouts. Moderate intensity refers to an activity that raises your heart rate and makes you breathe harder, while vigorous intensity involves a higher level of effort. Start with shorter sessions and gradually increase the duration as your fitness level improves. Aim for at least 150 minutes of moderate-intensity aerobic activity or 75 minutes of vigorous-intensity aerobic activity per week.

3. Interval Training: Consider incorporating interval training into your

cardio workouts. This involves alternating between periods of high-intensity exercise and active recovery. For example, alternate between sprinting and jogging. Interval training can help increase cardiovascular fitness, burn more calories, and improve endurance.

Strength and Resistance Training

Strength and resistance training are vital for building muscle strength, improving bone density, and boosting metabolism. Here are some key considerations for incorporating strength training into your fitness routine:

1. Exercise Selection: Choose exercises that target major muscle groups, such as squats, lunges, deadlifts, bench presses, shoulder presses, and rows. Include both compound exercises (those that work multiple muscle groups) and isolation exercises (targeting specific muscles).

2. Proper Form and Technique: Learn and practice proper form and technique for each exercise to ensure safety and effectiveness. Consider working with a fitness professional or personal coach to learn the correct form and avoid injuries.

3. Progressive Overload: Gradually increase the resistance or intensity of your strength training exercises over time. This principle of progressive overload stimulates muscle growth and strength gains. Use resistance equipment like dumbbells, barbells, resistance bands, or weight machines.

4. Frequency and Rest: Aim for two to three strength training sessions per week, allowing for at least 48 hours of rest between sessions targeting the same muscle group. This rest period allows muscles to recover and grow stronger.

Flexibility and Mobility Exercises

Flexibility and mobility exercises enhance joint range of motion, improve posture, and reduce the risk of injuries. Here are some points to consider:

1. Stretching: Incorporate static stretches that target major muscle groups after your workouts or on rest days. Hold each stretch for 15-30 seconds without bouncing or forcing the movement.

2. Dynamic Warm-up: Before engaging in any exercise, include dynamic warm-up exercises that involve moving joints and muscles through a full range of

motion. This prepares your body for activity and helps improve flexibility.

3. Yoga or Pilates: Consider participating in yoga or Pilates classes to improve flexibility, balance, and core strength. These disciplines often incorporate both stretching and strengthening exercises.

4. Mobility Drills: Include mobility drills that focus on specific joints or movement patterns to improve joint mobility and functional range of motion. Examples include hip circles, shoulder dislocations, or ankle mobility exercises.

Nutrition and Diet

Proper nutrition is crucial for fueling your body, supporting your fitness goals, and maintaining overall health and well-being. Understanding macronutrients and micronutrients, as well as developing a balanced and sustainable eating plan, are key components of a healthy diet.

Understanding Macronutrients and Micronutrients:

1. Macronutrients: Macronutrients are the three primary nutrients required in larger quantities for energy production and overall functioning of the body:

a. Carbohydrates: Carbohydrates are the body's primary source of energy. Include complex carbohydrates like whole grains, fruits, vegetables, and legumes in your diet. These provide fiber, vitamins, and minerals. Limit refined carbohydrates and sugary foods.

b. Proteins: Proteins are essential for building and repairing tissues, supporting muscle growth, and maintaining a healthy immune system. Include lean sources of protein such as poultry, fish, lean meats, dairy products, legumes, and plant-based protein sources like tofu and tempeh.

c. Fats: Healthy fats are necessary for hormone production, nutrient absorption, and providing energy. Include sources like avocados, nuts, seeds, fatty fish (such as salmon), olive oil, and coconut oil. Limit saturated and trans fats found in processed foods and fried items.

2. Micronutrients: Micronutrients are essential vitamins and minerals required in smaller quantities for various physiological functions:

a. Vitamins: Consume a variety of fruits, vegetables, whole grains, and lean proteins to obtain a broad range of vitamins, including vitamins A, C, D, E, and the B vitamins. These vitamins support energy production, immune function, and overall health.

b. Minerals: Include mineral-rich foods such as leafy greens, nuts, seeds, legumes, lean meats, and dairy products. Important minerals include calcium, iron, potassium, magnesium, and zinc, among others, which are necessary for proper bodily functions.

CHAPTER THREE

Developing a Balanced and Sustainable Eating Plan

1. Caloric Balance: Determine your caloric needs based on your goals, activity level, and body composition. Create a balance between caloric intake and expenditure to support your fitness goals (e.g., weight loss, maintenance, or muscle gain).

2. Whole Foods: Focus on consuming whole, minimally processed foods as the foundation of your diet. These foods are typically nutrient-dense, providing essential vitamins, minerals, and fiber

while avoiding excessive added sugars, unhealthy fats, and artificial additives.

3. Portion Control: Be mindful of portion sizes to ensure you're consuming appropriate amounts of each food group. Use measuring tools or visual cues (such as the size of your palm or a deck of cards) to estimate portion sizes.

4. Hydration: Stay adequately hydrated by drinking water throughout the day. Water supports digestion, nutrient absorption, and overall cellular

function. Avoid excessive intake of sugary beverages and alcohol.

5. Meal Planning: Plan your meals and snacks in advance to make healthier choices and avoid impulsive or unhealthy eating. Incorporate a balance of macronutrients and micronutrients in each meal, including lean proteins, whole grains, fruits, vegetables, and healthy fats.

6. Consistency and Sustainability: Focus on developing long-term eating habits that are sustainable and enjoyable. Avoid restrictive diets or extreme

approaches that are difficult to maintain. Consistency is key to achieving and maintaining optimal health and fitness.

Hydration and Its Impact on Fitness

Hydration is a crucial aspect of fitness and overall health. Proper hydration supports optimal physical performance, aids in temperature regulation, nutrient absorption, and promotes overall well-being. Here's why hydration is important and some tips to maintain adequate hydration:

1. Performance and Endurance: Dehydration can negatively impact

physical performance and endurance. Even mild dehydration can lead to reduced energy levels, fatigue, decreased concentration, and impaired cognitive function. Staying hydrated helps maintain optimal physical and mental performance during workouts or sports activities.

2. Temperature Regulation: Sweating is the body's natural mechanism for cooling down during exercise. Adequate hydration supports sweat production, which helps regulate body temperature. When you're dehydrated, your body may struggle to cool down efficiently,

leading to overheating and an increased risk of heat-related illnesses.

3. Nutrient Transport and Recovery: Water is essential for transporting nutrients, including carbohydrates, electrolytes, and oxygen, to the muscles. It also aids in the removal of waste products, such as lactic acid, which can accumulate during exercise. Proper hydration supports efficient nutrient transport and aids in post-workout recovery.

Tips for maintaining adequate hydration

- Drink water regularly throughout the day, even when you're not feeling thirsty. Thirst is not always an accurate indicator of hydration status.

- Monitor urine color. Aim for a pale yellow or straw-like color, which indicates proper hydration. Dark yellow urine may be a sign of dehydration.

- Consider your activity level and the environment. Increase fluid intake during intense workouts, hot weather, or high-altitude activities.

- Include hydrating foods in your diet, such as fruits and vegetables with high water content, like watermelon, cucumber, oranges, and strawberries.

- Carry a reusable water bottle with you to encourage regular hydration throughout the day.

- If engaging in prolonged or intense exercise, consider sports drinks that contain electrolytes to replenish lost fluids and minerals.

Finding the Right Personal Coach

A personal coach can provide guidance, motivation, and expertise to help you achieve your fitness goals. Here are some important qualities to look for when choosing a personal coach:

1. Certification and Credentials: Look for a coach who holds relevant certifications from reputable organizations. Common certifications include NASM (National Academy of Sports Medicine), ACE (American Council on Exercise), or ACSM (American College of Sports Medicine). These certifications indicate that the coach has met certain educational and professional standards.

2. Experience and Specialization: Consider the coach's experience in working with individuals with similar goals or conditions as yours. A coach with experience in your specific area of interest, whether it's weight loss, strength training, sports performance, or rehabilitation, can provide specialized guidance and support.

3. Communication and Motivational Skills: Effective communication is crucial for a successful coaching relationship. Look for a coach who listens attentively, communicates clearly, and understands your needs and preferences. A good

coach should be able to motivate and inspire you, providing positive reinforcement and support throughout your fitness journey.

4. Individualized Approach: A great coach will take the time to understand your unique needs, abilities, and limitations. They should develop personalized training programs that align with your goals, while also considering any health conditions or injuries you may have.

5. Adaptability and Flexibility: Fitness goals and circumstances can change over time. A coach who is adaptable

and willing to adjust your training plan accordingly is essential. They should be able to modify exercises, intensity, or duration as needed to accommodate your changing needs or circumstances.

6. Professionalism and Ethics: Look for a coach who maintains high professional standards and adheres to ethical guidelines. They should prioritize your safety, respect your boundaries, and maintain confidentiality.

CHAPTER FOUR

Designing a Well-Rounded Exercise Routine

A well-rounded exercise routine incorporates various components of fitness to ensure overall strength, endurance, flexibility, and balance. Consider the following components when designing your routine:

1. Cardiovascular Conditioning: Include activities that elevate your heart rate and improve cardiovascular fitness. Choose exercises that you enjoy and can sustain for a reasonable duration. Aim for at least 150 minutes of moderate-intensity aerobic activity or

75 minutes of vigorous-intensity aerobic activity per week.

2. Strength Training: Incorporate exercises that target major muscle groups to build strength and muscle mass. Use a combination of bodyweight exercises, free weights, resistance bands, or weight machines. Aim for two to three strength training sessions per week, allowing for rest and recovery between sessions.

3. Flexibility and Mobility: Dedicate time to stretching and mobility exercises to improve flexibility, joint range of

motion, and prevent injuries. Include static stretching after your workouts and consider activities like yoga or Pilates to enhance flexibility and mobility.

4. Balance and Stability: Include exercises that challenge your balance and improve stability, such as single-leg exercises, yoga poses, or balance boards. Developing balance and stability is essential for functional movements and injury prevention.

Adapting to Individual Fitness Levels and Abilities

Fitness programs should be adapted to individual fitness levels and abilities to ensure safety and effectiveness. Consider the following:

1. Modifications and Progressions: Tailor exercises to match your current fitness level. If an exercise is too challenging, modify it by using lighter weights, reducing the range of motion, or using assistance (e.g., resistance bands). As you progress, gradually increase the difficulty or intensity of exercises.

2. Listen to Your Body: Pay attention to your body's signals and adjust your workouts accordingly. If you experience pain or discomfort during an exercise, modify or stop the movement. Respect your body's limits and avoid pushing beyond what feels safe and manageable.

3. Seek Professional Guidance: If you're new to exercise or have specific health concerns or limitations, consider working with a fitness professional or personal coach. They can assess your fitness level, provide personalized guidance, and help you design a

program that suits your abilities and goals.

Remember that consistency and adherence to your fitness program are key to achieving results. Make sure to incorporate rest days for recovery and listen to your body's need for rest and recuperation.

Monitoring Progress

To ensure progress and make necessary adjustments, it's important to regularly monitor your metrics, track your body composition and fitness markers, and modify your training program accordingly. Here are some key considerations:

1. Measuring Body Composition and Fitness Markers:

a. Body Weight: Regularly monitor your body weight to track overall changes. However, keep in mind that weight alone doesn't provide a comprehensive picture of your progress, as it doesn't distinguish between fat and muscle mass.

b. Body Fat Percentage: Tracking your body fat percentage provides a more accurate reflection of changes in body composition. Methods such as skinfold calipers, bioelectrical impedance analysis (BIA), or

DEXA scans can help estimate body fat percentage.

c. Circumference Measurements: Measure key body circumferences, such as waist, hips, thighs, and arms, to monitor changes in body shape and fat distribution.

d. Fitness Markers: Track specific fitness markers relevant to your goals, such as cardiovascular endurance (e.g., time to complete a specific distance), strength (e.g., maximum weight lifted), flexibility (e.g., range of motion in specific stretches), or athletic performance (e.g., speed, agility).

2. Setting Realistic Milestones and Goals:

a. Short-Term Milestones: Break your long-term goals into smaller, achievable milestones. These milestones act as stepping stones towards your ultimate objective. For example, if your goal is to lose 20 pounds, set short-term milestones of losing 1-2 pounds per week.

b. SMART Goals: Ensure that your goals are Specific, Measurable, Achievable, Relevant, and Time-bound. This framework helps provide clarity and accountability to your objectives. For instance, a SMART goal could be "I will increase my maximum bench press by 10 pounds in 8 weeks."

c. Non-Scale Goals: It's important to set goals beyond just the numbers on the scale. Focus on non-scale victories such as increased energy levels, improved sleep quality, or the ability to perform exercises with better form or increased difficulty.

3. Modifying the Training Program as Needed:

a. Regular Assessment: Periodically reassess your progress and evaluate whether your current training program is still effective in helping you reach your goals. Consider reevaluating every 4-8 weeks, depending on your progress and the complexity of your goals.

b. Adjustments Based on Feedback: Pay attention to your body's response to the training program. If you consistently hit plateaus or experience lack of progress, it may be time to make adjustments. This could involve changing exercise selection, altering training volume or intensity, or incorporating new training techniques.

c. Gradual Progression: Gradually increase the challenge of your workouts over time to ensure continued progress. This can include increasing the weight lifted, adding more repetitions or sets, shortening rest periods, or incorporating more advanced exercises.

d. Periodization: Consider implementing a periodization approach to your training, which involves planned cycles of varying intensity and volume. This helps prevent plateaus, optimizes performance, and reduces the risk of overtraining.

e. Seek Professional Guidance: If you're unsure about how to modify your training program or track your progress effectively, consider consulting with a qualified fitness professional or personal coach. They can provide expert guidance, conduct assessments, and help you make appropriate adjustments.

Mental and Emotional Support

Achieving fitness goals requires more than just physical effort. It also involves developing a positive mindset, overcoming challenges, and staying motivated throughout the journey. Here are some strategies to support your mental and emotional well-being:

1. Developing a Positive Mindset:

a. Set Realistic Expectations: Avoid setting overly ambitious or unrealistic goals that may lead to frustration. Set goals that are challenging yet attainable, and celebrate each milestone achieved along the way.

b. Focus on Progress, Not Perfection: Recognize that progress is not always linear, and setbacks are a normal part of the process. Instead of dwelling on setbacks, focus on the progress you've made and the positive changes you've experienced.

c. Practice Positive Self-Talk: Replace negative self-talk with positive affirmations. Encourage yourself, acknowledge your efforts, and remind yourself of your capabilities. Reframe challenges as opportunities for growth.

d. Surround Yourself with Supportive People: Seek out individuals who encourage and support your fitness journey. Surrounding yourself with positive and like-minded individuals can provide motivation and accountability.

2. Dealing with Plateaus and Setbacks:

a. Reassess and Adjust: If you encounter a plateau or setback, take a step back and assess your current approach. Consider modifying your workout routine, adjusting your nutrition plan, or seeking guidance from fitness professional. Remember that plateaus are common, and with the right adjustments, progress can resume.

b. Set New Goals: Revisit and redefine your goals to keep yourself motivated. Setting new challenges or focusing on different aspects of fitness can reignite your enthusiasm and drive.

c. Find Inspiration: Seek inspiration from others who have overcome similar challenges or have achieved what you aspire to accomplish. Their success stories can serve as motivation and remind you that setbacks are temporary.

3. Incorporating Mindfulness and Stress Management Techniques:

a. Mindful Exercise: Practice mindfulness during your workouts by focusing on the present moment, tuning into your body, and fully experiencing the sensations of the activity. This can enhance your connection with your body, reduce stress, and improve overall well-being.

b. Stress Management: Engage in stress management techniques such as deep breathing exercises, meditation, yoga, or other relaxation techniques. These practices can help alleviate stress, improve mental clarity, and promote a sense of calm.

c. Balance and Self-Care: Ensure that your fitness routine allows for adequate rest and recovery. Prioritize sleep, engage in activities that you enjoy outside of fitness, and take time for self-care. Nurturing your overall well-being contributes to a positive mindset and sustained motivation.

d. Celebrate Non-Scale Victories: Focus on the non-scale victories and the positive changes you experience throughout your fitness journey. Celebrate improvements in energy levels, increased endurance, improved sleep quality, or enhanced self-confidence. Recognizing and acknowledging these achievements can boost motivation and self-esteem.

Remember that staying motivated and overcoming challenges is a personal journey. Find strategies that resonate with you and align with your values. It's normal to have ups and downs, but maintaining a positive mindset, seeking support, and implementing stress management techniques can help you navigate the challenges and stay motivated on your fitness journey.

CHAPTER FIVE

Taking Fitness Beyond Training

To make fitness a sustainable lifestyle choice, it's important to incorporate exercise into your daily life beyond structured training sessions. Here are some strategies to help you stay active and make fitness a seamless part of your everyday routine:

1. Active Living and Finding Opportunities for Movement:

a. Move Throughout the Day: Look for opportunities to incorporate movement into your daily activities. Take the stairs instead of the elevator, walk or bike to nearby destinations instead of driving, or schedule walking meetings instead of sitting in a conference room.

b. Break Sedentary Habits: If you have a sedentary job, take regular breaks to stretch, stand up, or do quick exercises like squats or lunges. Set reminders to get up and move every hour to counteract the negative effects of prolonged sitting.

c. Household Chores as Exercise: Engage in household chores that require physical exertion, such as cleaning, gardening, or DIY projects. These activities can contribute to your daily exercise quota while accomplishing necessary tasks.

d. Active Recreation: Choose recreational activities that involve movement and physical activity, such as hiking, dancing, swimming, or playing sports. These activities not only promote fitness but also provide enjoyment and a break from routine.

2. Incorporating Exercise into Work and Travel Routines:

a. Desk Exercises: Perform simple exercises discreetly at your desk, such as leg raises, desk push-ups, or seated stretches. These exercises can help counteract the negative effects of sitting for long periods and keep you energized.

b. Lunchtime or Midday Workouts: Utilize your lunch breaks or midday breaks for a quick workout. Whether it's a brisk walk, a gym session, or a yoga class, fitting in exercise during these breaks can refresh your mind and body.

c. Hotel Room Workouts: When traveling, make use of your hotel room for a workout. Bodyweight exercises, resistance bands, or portable exercise equipment can provide a convenient way to stay active even when you're away from home.

d. Explore Active Travel Options: When possible, opt for active transportation modes like walking or biking while traveling. Additionally, explore local fitness facilities or outdoor spaces for activities like hiking, jogging, or group fitness classes.

3. Making Fitness a Sustainable Lifestyle Choice:

a. Find Activities You Enjoy: Engage in physical activities that you genuinely enjoy. It could be dancing, swimming, playing a sport, or practicing martial arts. When you find activities you love, exercise becomes something you look forward to rather than a chore.

b. Set Realistic and Flexible Goals: Set goals that are achievable and adaptable to different circumstances. Flexibility allows you to adjust your fitness routine based on changing schedules, travel plans, or unforeseen events.

c. Accountability and Social Support: Find an exercise buddy or join group fitness classes to hold yourself accountable and stay motivated. Having a support system and exercising with like-minded individuals can make the experience more enjoyable and sustainable.

d. Prioritize Recovery and Rest: Allow your body adequate time to rest and recover. Overtraining can lead to burnout and injuries. Listen to your body, prioritize sleep, and include active recovery days or relaxation practices like yoga or meditation in your routine.

Integrating exercise into your daily life and making it a sustainable lifestyle choice requires a shift in mindset and a willingness to prioritize physical activity. By finding opportunities for movement, incorporating exercise into work and travel routines, and choosing activities you enjoy, you can seamlessly integrate fitness into your daily life, leading to long-term health and well-being.

Conclusion

Embracing fitness training and personal coaching can greatly enhance your journey towards long-term success in achieving your health and fitness goals. By understanding the importance of fitness training and the role of a personal coach, you can lay a solid foundation for your fitness journey. Incorporating essential components such as cardiovascular conditioning, strength and resistance training, and flexibility and mobility exercises ensures a well-rounded and balanced approach to fitness.

Nutrition and diet play a crucial role in fueling your body for optimal performance. Understanding macronutrients and micronutrients, as well as developing a balanced and sustainable eating plan, provides the necessary support for your fitness training.

Hydration, along with other lifestyle factors like sleeps and stress management, also significantly impacts your fitness journey. Finding the right personal coach with the right qualifications, experience, specialization, and effective communication and motivational skills is key to ensuring a positive and supportive coaching relationship.

Tailoring your fitness program to your individual needs and abilities maximizes results. Designing a well-rounded exercise routine that incorporates variety, progression, and adaptation to your fitness level ensures continued growth and improvement.

Monitoring your progress, tracking metrics, and adjusting your plan as needed are essential for staying on track. Measuring body composition and fitness markers, setting realistic milestones and goals, and modifying your training program when necessary help maintain momentum and motivation.

Overcoming challenges and staying motivated require a positive mindset and effective strategies. Incorporating mindfulness, stress management techniques, and seeking mental and emotional support help navigate plateaus and setbacks, ensuring long-term adherence to your fitness goals.

Taking fitness beyond training involves integrating exercise into your daily life. Embracing active living, incorporating exercise into work and travel routines, and making fitness a sustainable lifestyle choice enable you to maintain consistency and enjoy the benefits of a fit and healthy lifestyle.

In conclusion, by embracing fitness training and personal coaching, and integrating exercise into your daily life, you are setting yourself up for long-term success on your fitness journey. It's a commitment to your health and well-being that will positively impact your life in various aspects.

Remember to stay consistent, stay motivated, and prioritize your overall well-being as you strive towards your fitness goals.

THE END

www.ingramcontent.com/pod-product-compliance
Lightning Source LLC
Chambersburg PA
CBHW051914250726

48659CB00002B/654